Married to Lupus

MARY MAGDALENE JOHNSON-COLLINS

Copyright © 2022 Mary Magdalene Johnson-Collins
All rights reserved
First Edition

Fulton Books
Meadville, PA

Published by Fulton Books 2022

ISBN 978-1-63860-845-5 (paperback)
ISBN 978-1-63860-846-2 (digital)

Printed in the United States of America

To my loving (Late) husband Terrance Newkirk-Collins Jr.
Thank you!

Thank you for taking a chance on me despite the hands that we were dealt.

Thank you for the wounds that you dressed, for the hospital visits where you never complained, for those nights that you prayed me through my pain and made sure I smiled, even when I felt there was no reason to be happy.

Thank you to the man that God made just for me.

Thank you for giving me the will to fight, even when I wanted to give up.

Thank you for every Lupus walk you supported and every dream you made sure came true.

Thank you for your love, your kisses, your jokes, and our children.

Thank you for always making me feel beautiful.

I thank God every day, that he gave me a man that truly loved me; I never had to question your love.

It was always made sure that I felt it, even on our not-so-good days.

If I didn't tell you enough here on earth, I am shouting to the heavens.

Thank you, baby, I appreciate you! I will be fine, God has me.

Now, be my guardian angel until we meet again.

CHAPTER 1

Love at First Sight

Numbers 20:22—And whatsoever the unclean person toucheth shall be unclean; and the soul that toucheth it shall be unclean until even.

We first met when I was fifteen years old. Neither one of us knew who we were, but he was not afraid of me, nor was I flattered by him. We did not even know each other on a first-name basis. However, he had grown very fond of me, so I allowed him to get to know me. Some people will call it love at first sight, and I truly believe it was love at first sight for him, but it was not love at first sight for me. The years grew, and even though I was not as interested in him as he was in me, it did not seem to bother him.

He did everything in his power to get me to really notice him. At first, it was easy to hide, but soon after, I could no longer hide what appeared to be love for me, because he started appearing in places that were so noticeable even my family could see what this was truly doing to me. He began to show up in the most visible places; his favorite part of me was my body, and once again, I tried to ignore him, but I could not. So I just continued to act as if he didn't exist.

I think I was a little afraid at this point. Afraid of truly learning of him and discovering how deep down inside his love was for me. You see, I was not used to being with anyone, nor was I used to being involved with a man who had so much passion for me. So as time progressed, I felt like maybe instead of being afraid or pushing him away, I should go ahead and embrace him and allow him to love me as he was trying so hard to do.

So at fifteen years old, I opened my life to him and we began to date, but I had no idea what I was getting myself into. I really did not have anyone to talk to, and I did not feel that anyone would understand, anyway. I was really alone. It was at a very crucial time in my life, I had just lost my grandmother, my mom, and I were trying to rekindle a relationship that we really did not have. My dad was a workaholic, with his own family, and was nonexistent currently in my life. I felt like my girls would not understand. Hell, I barely understood what was happening to me.

My brother started noticing the change first. He would ask me questions about him, and I could not even give an answer because I could not truly explain who this person was or what he was doing to me. All I can tell you is that he chose me. He loved me, and I felt as if I had no choice but to choose him in return.

He had exposed himself to my life, and my body had accepted him without an open invitation. I considered the fact that maybe he was not so much for me to worry about, but I guess that was wrong. When you date someone, you truly get to know who they are and you never know what the outcome may be. When you choose just to go along with it and try to give people the benefit of the doubt, life can take a turn either for the best or the worst. In my case, I had no idea that I was headed for what would be considered the worst. No seat belt, no airbags, and no one to save me; it was just me.

CHAPTER 2

To Date or Not to Date?

Proverbs 16: 27—An ungodly man diggeth up evil: and in his lips, there is a burning fire.

On our first date, he was not so bad. He was quite inviting. A little shy but still knew how to make himself noticeable, but with respect. We had dated throughout high school, and now it was time for me to leave for college. I was so excited about going off to school. College was an exciting time in my life. I attended the amazing and beautiful Florida Memorial College, now known as Florida Memorial University. I had never been away from home before then, and I had no idea what to expect, but I was ready.

While I was there, I met some amazing individuals. I joined the astonishing ladies of Lambda Beta Chi Service Sorority Incorporated. The friends that I made became family, and life was just truly great at that moment. I had some stumbling blocks during this time of my life because, once again, we had some situations that took place with death, and I really did not know how to get past it.

There was also a time in my life when I was dating another guy and he was putting me through hell, so my life was a bit rough. I was diagnosed with PTSD and then, soon after, my best friend was attacked, and I thought I had had enough. So I chose to go home, not finishing my education, and once again, it took a toll on me. The decisions that I was making in my life at that time, I did not realize the outcome of, where it would lead me in the long run. At that time, I did not know God. Of course, I grew up in the church; I grew up knowing about prayer, knowing the Bible, and knowing this God that everyone was speaking of, but not really knowing who he was.

This little factor (which I considered small at that time) became a major factor of why I felt so alone. God was nowhere in my life, and I truly needed him.

I was truly lost in my life, still carrying on a relationship with somebody who made himself present but only at the times when I was at my lowest point in life. I did not know how to be alone, and I truly did not know how to get rid of him. Once again, I had no one to talk to; I just had to allow him to continue to be a part of my life, and I kept him a secret. I was truly depressed at this point of my life, so I decided to try life somewhere else. I packed up my things, left with one of my very good friends, and moved to Tallahassee, Florida.

Even with this move, I soon learned that with even being there, you could not run away from your problems. That also became a time when life really started to decline, and I went back home just as empty as I was before I left.

I started to work at a doctor's office and decided to leave this toxic relationship that I was in. I believe I only accepted what he gave because it was consistent. As a matter of fact, it was the only consistent thing I had going on at that time. I was holding on to someone who did not want me, and doing all this while still trying to find my purpose in this drama called life. However, my old flame was still coming around, a lot more, and I was allowing him to. I do not know if I had grown accustomed to his presence or if I was afraid to live without knowing he was there. You see, he was not so easy to walk away from. As a matter of fact, I would never be able to walk away from him.

CHAPTER 3

The Arranged Marriage

Proverbs 18:22—Whoso findeth a wife findeth a good thing, and obtaineth favour of the lord.

In 2011, my life changed forever. I had just given birth to my first child and first son on June 21, 2011. On December 27, 2011, I got married without my knowledge. Now I could properly introduce him to the world, because, after all these years, I finally had a name to this man that had so much control over my life. His name was lupus. Discoid lupus, to be exact. I did my research to get to know him better (you would think by now that I knew him well), but unfortunately, I did not know what he was capable of.

At this time, he was really coming out for everyone to see, and even though my family had met him once before, they were really just then getting a true feel of who he really was. He was no longer just in my ears anymore, because remember, I told you he loved my body; he had taken complete control over my scalp. You see, I felt like this was an unfair situation because, as I stated in the beginning, I had just had a baby, and at that time, he was only six months old. I began to feel very angry with myself because had I not opened my life to him and allowed this person to enter it, then maybe I would have had a chance.

When I look back to those days, I realize I really did not have a choice. He had already entered my life without my knowledge and my consent. Not only did he date me without my even dating him first, but he had also now arranged for us to be together for the rest of our lives. Now I understand the feeling of an arranged marriage. Being forced to be with someone that you truly do not know. And to be frank, he was so aggressive and so consistent that I was afraid. His love for me was a love I was not sure I was ready for. Or that I even wanted. In the beginning, I felt like he had respect for me, even though I showed no interest in him. He at least still showed me some kindness, because he only stayed in one area of my body. But I guess he felt he had something to claim; just being in one restricted area was not enough for him. He wanted the world to know who he was, and he wanted the world to know whom I belonged to. Therefore, by his attaching himself to me and placing himself where everyone could see, I would be forced to expose him. I started to see that he loved the attention. But I did not. This was not a choice that I made for myself, and the worst part about it for me was, I had no way to get out. I was stuck, lost, scared, and now married and unable to escape. We were bonded for the rest of our lives.

Till death do us part.

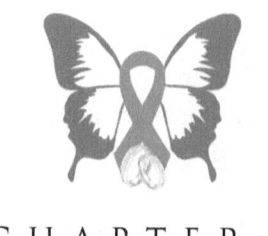

CHAPTER 4

The Vows

Genesis 3:24—Therefore shall a man leave his father and mother and shall cleave unto his wife: and they shall be one flesh.

"To have and to hold, for better or for worse, in sickness and in health, until death do us part."

To have and to hold—for a couple to be joined as one (my ears).

For better or for worse—sticking it out with each other through thick and thin no matter the outcome (my scalp).

In sickness and in health—by any means necessary (my body).

Till death do us part—control (my life).

The vows for me were different. And when you say them out loud, they hit differently.

For him, he thought he had full control over me, and the sad truth is, he did. He was beating me left and right, and I was taking it. Every hit, every ugly word, every harsh lash. I took it. I had no clue what marriage was, and I was so depressed and unhappy. One thing that I did not know at that time was that the lower I became in my emotions, the easier it made for lupus to take over my life. My body was declining faster, and I was in and out of the hospital monthly.

During this time, I met a man. Yeah, I allowed someone to come into this life of mine and all its craziness. I didn't feel that I was equipped to have him in my life due to everything that was taking place, but he refused to give up.

In November of 2012, we started dating. I was still 180 pounds and had most of my hair; I was able to get hairstyles to cover the discoid lupus so that he could not see the damage from my relationship. I was able to still be Mary without feeling so unattractive. I wasn't sure if the man I had chosen to be with at that time could handle everything that I was really going though, so when we started to get very serious, I was very blunt. My words to him were, "Look! I have lupus, as you can see. I am always in and out of the hospital. Unfortunately, this is my life. If you are planning on being here, this is what it is. You are *not* obligated to be here and deal with this. So at any even given time that you feel you want to walk away, you may do so and it will not hurt my feelings."

Whoa, Mary! I know. The blessed thing about this was, he took it. My bluntness, my attitude, my hurt, my depression, my hospital visits, my *everything*! He not only accepted it, but he also chose to stay.

In 2013, Terrance Collins asked Mary Magdalene Johnson to be his wife, and for once in her life, she knew what was best for her life and she said yes. Now, where was life going to take us from this day forth? We had no clue, but one thing he assured me of was, he was here for the ride.

CHAPTER 5

Loneliness

Mark 15:34—On the cross, He cried out, "My God, my God, why have you forsaken me?"

March 8, 2015, Terrance and I became husband and wife. We had no clue what marriage was all about or what vows we were about to be tested with. Sickness and health made sure we were introduced right at the start. I had become sick right before we got married. I was even thinking about taking a leave from work. But what kind of look would that have been to take a sick leave but still have a wedding? I know, worried about what people would say and how I would look in the process.

These were also reasons I was sick so often. Stress played a significant factor in my life. By the time we were wedded, I was 196 pounds. On sixty milligrams of prednisone every day and six other medications that I cannot even pronounce. And I was tired. Mentally exhausted and trying my hardest not to give up.

I was admitted into Bethesda Hospital on May 21, 2015, due to numbness on my left side. I had gotten up to walk to the bathroom and could not stand on my feet. I called out for Terrance because I was terrified and not sure what the heck was going on with me. As he awoke, by then my legs were so big and I had no feeling on my left side. From shoulder down to my foot, everything was numb, and

I was in a great deal of pain. I had my husband go ahead and pack a bag because I just knew they were going to keep me.

We left for the hospital—I refused to go by ambulance. I believe we both were very scared this time around because this was something new. Once we arrived at Bethesda, they took me to the back right away, checked my vitals, and contacted my doctor. It was not even ten minutes and already they were taking me to the back and I was placed into a room. Still terrified and in so much pain, I waited patiently, not realizing what was happening. Currently, I was experiencing pain, swelling, numbness, and tingling.

I was having a stroke.

Twenty-nine years old and having a stroke. *Are you kidding me, Mary?* This was ridiculous and unacceptable. I refused to allow something that I did not even choose to come into my life and take my life from me. I needed to fight, and I vowed to myself that I was going to fight or die trying. During this time of being in the hospital, I went through so many tests, and my doctor decided to bring in a few more amazing doctors to help him try to pinpoint what was going on with my body. I was still in a great deal of pain five days later, and we still had no answers.

On May 26, 2015, after seeing my primary cardiologist, neurologist, and rheumatologist, I was over it. No one could give me the answers that I needed. I was not going to continue down this road. I felt bad for my doctors, though; they had to look me in the face and tell me they had no clue what was wrong or why this was happening. At that moment, I made the choice to go home. I talked it over with my doctor, and he allowed me to discharge myself, and I did.

I went home the same way I came, and mentally that placed me in a state of depression that I had never been in before. I was devastated, and I felt more alone. You see, people feel they can help with their words; however, sometimes people need to keep their words to themselves when it comes to things that they cannot truly help with. I had individuals in my life, family members and friends who I knew meant well, but the way their words were given, they could have kindly kept them in their thoughts. To be fair to them, being sick is like having a death happen, and all people can do and say is,

"I am sorry for your loss." We, as human beings, say this because this is what we have been taught to say, but what do those words help? Nothing. Does it really give comfort to the person who has lost someone? No, no, it does not. After a while, you get tired of hearing it, and for some, they just shut down. This was how my loneliness felt; I could not talk to anyone but God, and this was when I knew it was time.

CHAPTER 6

Exit Plan

Proverbs 18: 21—Death and life are in the power of the tongue: and they that love it shall eat the fruit thereof.

Life as I knew it then had changed, and I was going home a different woman. I had to get away from him, and I was ready. I was leaving this place with a different mindset, and I was planning my exit plan; I was going to be free from lupus. I did not know just how I was going to do this just yet, but I had a few ideas that I was going to try, and I was determined.

Now, no disrespect to the medical world, but if I could not get any answers from those that were treating me, then it was time to go home and be one with the one who created me. I was going home to find Jesus. It was time to get on one accord with God and heal this body that he made.

I went home on more medication, and I was not taking it. As a matter of fact, I had my mind made up that I was not taking any more of that crap. Now, for those of you who are reading this book, do not—and I repeat, do *not*—stop taking your medication. Before you decide to do anything, consult with your doctor first! I had given up on the medical world, so the choices that I was about to take, I was ready for the consequences of the results of my actions. So I stopped all my meds at one time. Cold turkey. And I did not tell a soul. Not my husband, not my mom, not my best friends, not anybody. Reasons were, again, that no one felt what I felt and they could not understand what I was going through. Also, I was tired of being a guinea pig for the medical world. Yes, I said it! This is how a lot of lupus patients feel; hell, this how a lot of us with autoimmune diseases feel. We are science experiments for new medications, trial and error to see what will work on us, not work at all, or kill us off. But remember, these are my personal thoughts, how I felt at that very moment, and I was not ready to die.

So what was I planning on doing about it? Once I stopped taking meds, what was my plan? The sad part was, I had no idea; I just knew I needed to get away. I did not even have a clue as to how my body would react to just getting off my meds. Well, I was about to find out, and this had to truly be one of the scariest days of my life.

I came home from work early one day. Kamden was in aftercare, so I did not have to bring him home with me, and my husband was at work. I came home to an empty house, and I was sick as a dog. At first, I had no idea what was going on with me until after my head had been in the toilet of our master bathroom for over an hour. I was detoxing. I had chills and sweats. I was vomiting and unable to get off the floor. I was not sure what death felt like, but boy, when I tell you, I would not wish this feeling for my worst enemy. All I can remember me saying is, "Lord God, if you allow me to get through this, I promise I will not do anything this stupid again. Please just don't let me die."

Remember, I was alone. There was no one home with me. No one knew that I was off my medication. No one knew I had gone back home sick, and if I had died, my husband would have come home to a wife who was no longer here because of a selfish choice that she decided to make on herself. That was the day I met God for myself in a whole new way. Not in a church, not from a person of faith, but on my own, in my home, on the bathroom floor, dying. But he let me live.

That was the day I gave my life to Christ, and I mean *really* gave my life to Christ, and I would not change anything about it. This is my testimony and the day he gave me a new life. For this, I am thankful, and for this, he gave me my exit plan away from this life that had chosen me.

For the first time in a long time, I felt as if I was free. I was no longer attached to this thing; I was able to let go and truly let God. Break out from this marriage as I felt it was and move on with freedom.

I did not know what life was going to be without my medication or lupus, but I did not care. Anything was better than what I was dealing with every day. No more abuse, no more losing my hair, no more fatigued days, no more swelling, no more of this disease taking over my life. I was getting my life back, and I no longer felt alone, because I had a doctor who could do what man could not. It was time to escape; my bags were back, and I was gone. Thank you, Jesus! I was finally free.

CHAPTER 7

Making Uncomfortable Changes

Galatians 5:1—Stand fast therefore in the liberty wherewith Christ hath made us free, and be not entangled again with the yoke of bondage.

Freedom felt great, but it came with some changes that I had to be willing to endure. I had to leave what I loved the most, and that was my job, my department, my kids. I cried like a baby; the last thing I wanted to do was to come out of the classroom, but I did not have a choice. I had to leave all stress behind me, and I had to let it go so that I could get better. However, coming out of the classroom meant having to take a pay cut. My husband was still in school at that time, and money was already tight. We had to sacrifice a lot for this journey but God.

We ended up moving back in with my mom and letting our apartment go. It was so heartbreaking, but it was what had to be done until I was in a better state of health. I commend my baby in this area, because for a man to suck up his pride and make a move such as the one I was asking of him showed me just who my husband really was. A remarkable man who stood right by his wife's side during a very tough time in her life. And he did unselfishly. This showed me just how much he loved me. I knew these choices that we were making did indeed come with some major ups and downs. I had to find a new job position, change schools, travel back and forth for Kamden due to not wanting to uproot him from his school and friends, and still try to make this pay cut work for these bills. All I kept asking myself was, Are you sure you are making the right choice, Mary? Why not just take the meds and find another way? But that was not what I wanted, and so I did not. I was not aware at that very moment, but I was learning about faith and had no idea what faith was. Whether or not I was ready to learn this lesson, I am pretty sure that this was also a part of the changes that I needed to make. To fully trust and believe that God has this all under control. To just have faith.

I called one of my best friends over to the house one night, and we talked, laughed, and hung out like old times. Then I asked her to do something that I still, to this day, do not feel she was comfortable with doing, but she did it for me. I asked her to cut my hair. To cut it all off. This was the next phase of the process.

I felt like for this to really be real to me, I needed to heal my wounds. God was teaching me how to heal the inner soul of my body, so I needed to heal the outer scars that depressed me. So she agreed. As she cut my hair, she cried, and I assured her it was okay. But I was also dying on the inside. I was grateful for her, and she did not even know. She was doing something for me that I did not have the guts to do on my own. God knew I needed her at that moment.

Once she finished, we cried together, but again, I was free. I then asked my uncle to cut my hair down to a fade because I needed to see every spot. I needed to confront everything that made me feel defeated, and my hair was a major one. Lupus might have taken it from me, but I was determined to get me back. All of me.

(Let the cutting begin and let us see the damage!)

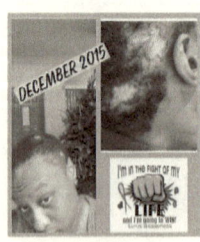

CHAPTER 8

Lessons to Be Learned

Psalms 103:2–3—Bless the LORD, O my soul, And forget not all his benefits: Who forgiveth all thine iniquities; Who healeth all thy diseases.

Okay, guys, now, as you know, I have stepped out on faith and I am healing my scars. So what does this mean for me? I am filing for a divorce from lupus. See, it is one thing for one to be joined without say, but it is another to be able to leave and leave legally with say. How do you divorce a disease? Well, to be honest, I was not born with this. So how did I end up with lupus in the first place? The only thing I could think of was, there was a shift somewhere in my body that caused this to happen. Though things happen without our control, we can do research and fix what is broken. So what did I do? I took back my life by changing my eating habits. I decided to stop eating pork, beef, and sweets. I made a choice to let go of all processed food and canned goods. What did this mean for me? More changes, lessons that I was learning about my body. I had no idea what I was doing to my body. Or had done.

As children, we eat what our parents and caregivers give us. We do not question, for we are grateful for the food on our tables. But whether our children like it or not, we need to do a little better with what we serve on our tables. I found out that a lot of the things that I had been eating over the years were a significant factor of why my body was failing and how I ended up married to lupus in the first place. He was literally handed to me on a plate with a silver spoon. This was how I received him without knowledge, and there was no one to blame; it was a lesson learned.

Now, how was I sure that this was the cause of the problem? I chose one day to get up and go have colonic done. I figured, before I started the next phase of my journey, I needed to cleanse out what had been packed down in my body for twenty-seven years. I do not know why this is something we do not do regularly throughout our lives. Our bodies need to release what we place inside of them, which is why we poop (laughing at the obvious). So why are we not properly cleaning out our intestines? I got up one morning and decided today would be the day to go and get one done. I had taken a detox tea for five days before I made the choice to go so that I could get a head start in cleaning out my body. I thought, by doing this, my experience would be a great one, because I would not have much to clean out. Well, let us just say, if you have never had one done, I really recommend it to everyone. It was the best experience I have ever had, and it allowed me to see just how backed up my body was. I was embarrassed and ashamed that I had waited so long before doing something like this for my body. It took seven flushes until I was finally seeing clear fluids from my intestines (sorry if that sounds gross), but this shows you all why this is important.

Now that I had reached this part of the journey, this must be the end, right? Was this what it took just to say that I was finally free? No, not at all. This was just the beginning, and I was well on my way, with still a long way to go. One of the major lessons learned here was how to treat my body, protect my body, and remember that my body is a temple. You only get one, and you need to treat it as such.

Lesson learned.

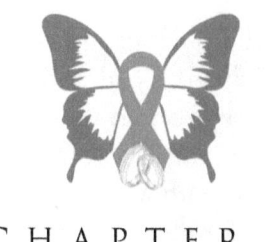

CHAPTER 9

Juicing to Live

Jeremiah 33:6—Behold, I will bring it health and cure, and I will cure them, and will reveal unto them the abundance of peace and truth.

Fruits and vegetables are good for you; eat them every day so you can grow up healthy and smart. Right? I think so. What is better than veggies? Green veggies! Terrance and I decided to further this journey, and we went shopping for a juicer. This was a very hard part for me because I am one who loves to eat. Not being able to have the things that I wanted and craved for was where I knew I had to heal mentally. I had to constantly remind myself this was for my own good, and in order for me to heal, I had to change my mental state as well.

We started to look up different juicing recipes, and I even had my other bestie and her husband to join us. We shared recipes, which made this a little easier and more enjoyable. Once I got to this part of the journey, I started to feel so much better. We had been trying to have a baby also, but with so much going on, I was told that I would not be able to have any more kids, so we gave up on that dream and just focused on my getting better and healing from the inside out.

For once, I was focused, exercising, and eating better. This was an amazing feeling for me. I had not felt this good in so long, and for once in my life, I had not been in anyone's hospital in eleven months! It was now May 2016, and life took a turn for a moment.

I was admitted into the hospital for hidradenitis suppurativa. I was so bummed but relieved that this had nothing to do with my lupus. I am not sure why this came about, but it did, and it could have been because of all the cleaning I was doing; I am not sure, but it happened. I will not go in-depth with this, but let's just say that once again I was out of work for almost five months. I had to exhaust my 401(k) just so we did not lose what we had just built back up. Working on one's mental state when you're working on your health and having both of them fighting you back at the same time is not fun. I was trying so hard to stay positive, but I am not going to lie—I was feeling so defeated.

How can one feel defeated when you have God on your side? Well, that is easy to answer. When you are trying to do things on your own and not seeking his guidance, it is easy to get low and back to the place you were just released from. I had chosen to live! I was now juicing and eating better because I wanted to live. But I was forgetting that this might have started off being about freeing myself from something that thought it could take me away. However, it was much bigger than that. In order to truly live, I had to do more than just what I was doing; there was more to this journey, much more. I needed to not only juice to live but also heal and trust God. This process was what I truly needed. We all did.

CHAPTER 10

Healing and Trusting God

Ephesians 6: 10–13—Finally, my brethren, be strong in the Lord, and in the power of his might. Put on the whole armour of God, that ye may be able to stand against the wiles of the devil. For we wrestle not against flesh and blood, but against principalities, against powers, against the rulers of the darkness of this world, against spiritual wickedness in high places. Wherefore take unto you the whole armour of God, that ye may be able to withstand in the evil day, and having done all, to stand.

As life continued for me, we really hit some very rough bumps. My health, our marriage, our jobs, just life in general. I needed a church home, and I did not have one. I refused to go back to my church, and my husband's church just did not do it for me. I needed a place where my spirit would be fed. You see, with having lupus, it also brings about depression, insomnia, and anxiety. I do not care how much medication they make in the world; nothing can get you past these three things better than God. This, too, was a part of my healing process, and I was struggling because with these spirits comes fighting time. I couldn't fight something that I was not equipped to battle on my own. I had given my life to God, but what now? Healing took more than just changing what I ate and running away from this place of my life that I hated so much. I hated lupus with a passion, and I know hate is such a strong word, but that was how I felt. This was hatred I was still carrying around with me. I would not even speak his name because I felt like if I did at any given moment, I would invite him back into my life, and I could not do that to myself again. I know, that's crazy, right? When you are healing, you need to be willing to change everything. One needs to release hate, fear, nervousness, etc., anything that still ties you to what you're trying to get away from. Lupus had me mentally even though I was healing. This was where I was still struggling, and God was my only hope of releasing it all. This was where he blessed me more than he knew, or shall I say, more than I thought he would.

I set out and started my journey to find a place for me and my family. I decided to search around until I found one. I was not comfortable with church hopping. I was not having any luck on my own, so I cried out once again for God to guide me on finding a place where I would be fed, that my husband would like, and that Kamden would be willing to go to without having to fight with him about it. By his blessings, he sent us Christ Fellowship. From the first time I walked into the building, I knew I was at home. My family left that day more than satisfied; we were overly blessed. This is the day I am most thankful for, and I will always be. Learning to trust God in the midst of my storm was what was the most important part of healing from this illness, from this arranged marriage. God gave me so much; he was not finished with me yet, though. I just did not know how well he listens to my cries.

CHAPTER 11

But God

Jeremiah 17:7—Blessed is the man that trusteth in the Lord, and whose hope the Lord is.

In October of 2016, I became pregnant. Remember, I was told I could not have any more children. But God, I prayed and asked God to give my husband and my son their wish. I knew Terrance wanted a child of his own, and both he and Kamden wanted a girl. I asked God if he would please do this for me. I would be so grateful if he did. And just like that, he answered my prayers. Not only did my God give my husband a child, but he also gave him a girl. Now, the funny part about this was, my son had laid his hand on my belly one night and said his own prayer for his baby sister. And guess what? God also answered his prayers too (ha!). Isn't God amazing? Honey, let me tell you, this was just the beginning of life changing for us. Of course, now, when things are going well, something always must come in and try to destroy the blessing.

    I had set out to have a home birth. I felt deep down that this would be hard for me because I knew that the moment I told a physician that I had lupus, they were going to turn me away or tell me that a home birth was not an option. So here we go again, feeling some defeat, but trying so hard to stay positive. Let me go back to when I gave birth to Kamden. It wasn't until six months later that I was diagnosed, so was this going to be the same way, or was it going to get worse? Here I was, worrying again when I was supposed to be trusting God, right? Right! So I told myself that I would keep searching until I found the right doctor for me. I thought I had her until she backed out on me also. I had a high-risk doctor, and he wanted me to be on a baby aspirin just in case something happened, and I refused that as well. I was not on any medications, and I was not going to take any baby aspirin or whatever for a problem that was non-existence in my life. Yes, I know, I sounded very disobedient, but I was not dropping my guns. My goal was to have this child the way God intended. I was going to have a natural birth if my life depended on it, and I was not taking no for an answer. Well, I was alone again. No doctor and due to give birth in three weeks. Ha! Yes, I said it, three weeks, and I had no doctor, you guys. It was really me and God. I was prepared that if I had to wait until my water broke and just give birth at any hospital that would take me, that was what I was going to do. Once again, I was being stubborn, but this time, I knew who God was, and I knew I would be fine.

Then he did what I knew he would: he sent me Kathy, my amazing midwife, and she gave me a chance. I was very honest with her and her backup doctor, and they were amazing to me. I love her because she gave me my hope back, and just like once again, I had beaten lupus another round! On July 13, at 10:32 p.m., Kennedi T. Collins was born, and I not only had her naturally but also had a VBAC. But God!

CHAPTER 12

Faith

Hebrews 11:1—Faith is being sure of what you hope for and certain of what you do not see.

Today I can write this book to give someone else like me faith and hope. No, you may not be able to see what is at the end of the tunnel, but have faith that God has your back and it will be a bright, amazing light waiting in your victory.

I lost sight of my light a few times, but each time God led me back to where I was able to have victory on my journey. Please do not give up or let this illness, or any illness, steal away who you are meant to become. Fight until you cannot fight anymore. This was what I had chosen to do, fight. I just knew this was not the end of the road for me. I knew God had bigger and better plans for me. I trusted and believed in that, and I always will. I pray the way I designed this book will give you all a picture of all I endured. I know some others that are battling lupus have gone through far worse than I have. But each journey for all of us is so different, and sometimes we do not know if we are coming or going.

For me, this is more than a book; this is hope. This is my way to finally say I am free, and I can now announce to the world that I am healed. Here I am in May of 2020. Levels are great, blood work is great, and I am still on no medications.

I am finally free!

www.ingramcontent.com/pod-product-compliance
Lightning Source LLC
Chambersburg PA
CBHW021000180526
45163CB00006B/2446